MY DIET
MY HAPPINESS

Towards a more nourished, longer, healthier and ultimately happier life

Enai Andres

Introduction

In the hustle and bustle of modern life, where the demands of work, family, and countless responsibilities seem to pull us in every direction, one fundamental aspect that have a significant impact on our overall well-being is our relationship with food. "My Diet My Happiness" is more than just a guide to proper nutrition. It explores the complex dance between our diet, physical health, and the elusive pursuit of true happiness. This book is not about hard rules, quick fixes, or one-size-fits-all solutions. Instead, we take you on a journey of self-discovery, encouraging you to listen to your body, understand your personal nutritional needs, and develop a positive, sustainable relationship with food.

We delve into the science of nutrition, the psychology of eating, and the profound impact that eating habits have on our physical and mental health. The author explains the trials and tribulations of figuring out the confusing nutritional advice, interpreting the signals of a unique body and embracing the happiness that comes from a harmonious relationship with oneself through accessible anecdotes, scientific discoveries and practical wisdom. But this journey isn't just physical, it's about understanding the deep connection between what we eat and how we feel. Our diet affects not only our weight and energy levels, but also our mood, mental clarity, and overall sense of well-being.

The purpose of this book is to explore the interplay between nutrition and emotion so that you can make choices that not only nourish your body but also contribute to a more enjoyable and fulfilling life. From practical tips on mindful eating to insightful anecdotes of people who changed their lives by changing their diet, this book will help you build a sustainable, balanced, and enjoyable relationship with food. The pages that follow are a call to reconsider our decisions, acknowledge our successes and draw lessons from our failures. We are urged to accept the ability we possess to mold our lives and create a genuine, balanced and eternally joyful experience as we turn the pages.

So, let the journey begin—a journey that promises not just the transformation of our bodies but the enrichment of our souls, a journey toward a life where diet, health and happiness converge in a symphony of well-being. Embark on this journey with an open mind and curiosity, and explore the transformative power of conscious nutrition on your path to lasting health and happiness.

Chapter 1

A Trip Down Memory Lane

It can be intriguing to take a trip down memory lane and investigate the food factors that molded your eating patterns and nutritional knowledge. You might be able to understand how your upbringing influenced your relationship with food by thinking back on these factors.

It's crucial to consider your family and cultural backgrounds while starting a new culinary endeavor. Did you have your upbringing in a particular ethnic or cultural background with its own distinct food and eating customs? Our early homes are frequently a mingling pot of influences from many eras and backgrounds, all of which shape the way we think about eating.

Next, think about how your family has influenced the way you eat. Family meals were important in your youth, especially if your parents or grandparents were good cooks. Their food choices, cooking methods and recipes can have a big impact on how you think about and approach nutrition.

In addition, looking at the kinds of meals that were popular when you were a child can provide insightful information. In your home, were prepared meals or processed foods more prevalent? Did you always include fresh fruits and veggies in your meals, or did you make them less of an emphasis? Examining these variables can help you have a better comprehension of the dietary principles you were taught growing up.

Exposure to various cuisines and culinary experiences outside of your household is another aspect to take into account. Did your friends and peers encourage you to try different meals and cuisines, or did you get the chance to sample them on family vacations or in ethnic restaurants? One's palate can be expanded, new flavors and foods can be tried and these encounters may have an impact on what they eat in the future.

Lastly, it's important to think back on the dietary education and information you received as a child. Regarding the significance of well-balanced meals, appropriate portion sizes and the nutritional worth of various foods, did you receive any official instruction or guidance? One's eating choices and long-term health can be significantly impacted by their understanding of the scientific aspects of nutrition.

Chapter 2
The Quest of a Healthy Life

The quest of a healthy, well-balanced diet is more important than ever in our fast-paced, modern life. Our dietary decisions affect not just our physical health but also our mental and physical well-being, vitality and energy levels. This chapter takes you on a journey to discover the complex interplay of tastes, nutrients and lifestyle choices that go into creating a truly nourishing way of living. It attempts to provide clarity and direction on the essential elements that make up a healthy, balanced diet in a world full of contradictory dietary advice and fast fixes. We will examine the necessary nutrients and the science underlying their function from the macro to the micro. From the macro to the micro, we will explore the essential nutrients, the science behind their roles in the body and the art of crafting meals that not only satiate our hunger but also fuel our lives with vitality.

Diving into the pages, you will discover the significance of macronutrients like proteins, carbohydrates and fats, as well as the vital role micronutrients play in supporting various bodily functions. We will explore the power of antioxidants, delve into the world of vitamins and minerals and uncover the secrets of maintaining a healthy relationship with food.

Beyond the realms of nutrition, you will find the cultural, social and psychological aspects of eating and explore the importance of mindful eating, the impact of food choices on the environment and the joy that can be found in savoring the diverse flavors that our world has to offer. In this chapter, we will explore the intricate web of nutrition, shedding light on the various components that make up a balanced and wholesome diet. Just as a maze has multiple paths leading to different destinations, the world of nutrition offers a plethora of dietary options, each claiming to hold the key to optimal health and happiness. **Let's get started:**

The Building Blocks of Nutrition: Our bodies are intricate machines that require the right fuel to function optimally. To understand how nutrition plays a pivotal role in our well-being, we must first grasp the fundamental building blocks of our diet. From macronutrients such as carbohydrates, proteins and fats to micronutrients like vitamins and minerals, each plays a unique role in supporting our bodily functions.

Personalizing Your Plate: Just as each path in a maze caters to different preferences, dietary choices should be tailored to individual needs and goals. Personalize nutrition – acknowledging that one size does not fit all, and explore various dietary patterns, from plant-based to Mediterranean.

Nutrient-rich diet: To ensure a wide range of nutrients, include a variety of whole foods, including fruits, vegetables, whole grains, lean proteins, and healthy fats.

Balance: Aim for a balanced intake of macronutrients (carbohydrates, proteins, fats) and micronutrients (vitamins, minerals).

Mindful Eating: Pay attention to your hunger and fullness signals and eat consciously instead of on autopilot.

Enjoyment: Enjoy the flavor and texture of food and promote a positive relationship with food.

Water Intake: Water is essential for many bodily functions such as digestion, nutrient absorption, and temperature regulation, so make sure you stay properly hydrated.

Physical Activity: Incorporate regular exercise according to your preferences and abilities to improve your physical and mental health.

Sleep: Prioritize proper, quality sleep as it is important for your overall health and rest.

Cooking Discovery: Learn how to prepare nutritious meals at home and gain more control over ingredients and cooking methods.

Flavor Enhancement: Experiment with herbs, spices, and healthy cooking techniques to enhance the flavor of your meals.

Social and Cultural Influences: Maintain social connections and share meals with others to foster a sense of community and support.

Cultural Considerations: Embrace the positive aspects of cultural dietary traditions and incorporate them into your diet.

Emotional Well-Being: Develop effective stress management strategies such as mindfulness, meditation, and hobbies to maintain emotional balance.

Positive Relationships: Maintain healthy relationships and surround yourself with a positive social environment.

Educational Awareness: Nutrition Knowledge: Stay informed about nutrition and adapt your decisions based on evidence-based information.

Lifelong Learning: Promote an attitude of continuous learning, staying open to new information and adapting your lifestyle accordingly.

Chapter 3
Challenges and Choices that Impact Diet

The modern world offers us an unparalleled array of options, ranging from conventional diets to the newest trends in nutrition, each with their own benefits and drawbacks. It becomes a delicate dance to strike a balance between the demands of a fast-paced lifestyle and the desire for a healthy diet, one that is complicated by time limits, contradicting information and the appeal of convenience. Along the way, we address issues that go beyond simple dietary choices and explore the fundamentals of our connection with food and how it affects our bodies and brains.

The goal of this chapter is to simplify the complex web of decisions and difficulties that overlap with diet and health. We hope to shed light on the complex interplay between our choices and the repercussions they have on the whole picture of our wellbeing by carefully examining scientific discoveries, individual stories and cultural influences. Come along with us as we set out on a life-changing journey that involves navigating the maze of food decisions and health issues that affect how we live.

Certainly! People often face various challenges and choices that can significantly impact their diet.

Here are some common challenges and choices that individuals may encounter:

Time Constraints: Challenge: Busy schedules and lack of time may lead to choosing convenient but less nutritious food options.

Choice: Prioritizing meal planning, preparation and choosing quick yet healthy options can help overcome this challenge.

Social influences: Social events and gatherings may involve unhealthy food choices.

Choice: Making conscious decisions about portion control, selecting healthier options, or bringing nutritious alternatives to social events can be empowering.

Emotional Eating Challenge: Emotional stress or boredom may lead to unhealthy eating habits.

Choice: Developing alternative coping mechanisms, such as exercise, mindfulness, or seeking support, can help break the cycle of emotional eating.

Nutritional Knowledge: Lack of understanding about nutrition may result in poor food choices.

Choice: Investing time in learning about nutrition, reading labels and seeking guidance from health professionals can enhance nutritional awareness.

Budget Constraints: Limited financial resources may make it challenging to afford healthier food options.

Choice: Identifying cost-effective yet nutritious foods, buying in bulk and planning meals ahead can help manage a tight budget.

Cultural and Dietary preference: Balancing cultural or personal dietary preferences with nutritional needs can be challenging.

Choice: Finding creative ways to incorporate traditional foods into a balanced diet and exploring diverse, healthy recipes can help strike a balance.

Health Conditions: certain health conditions may require dietary restrictions.

Choice: Seeking guidance from healthcare professionals, following prescribed dietary guidelines and making informed choices that align with health needs are crucial in managing such challenges.

Marketing and Food Advertising: Exposure to persuasive food marketing may influence unhealthy choices.

Choice: Developing media literacy skills, critically evaluating marketing messages and making conscious decisions about food purchases can counteract the impact of marketing.

Lifestyle Changes: Changes in lifestyle, such as a new job or relocation, can disrupt established eating habits.

Choice: Adapting and planning for these changes, maintaining a routine and being mindful of food choices during transitions can help mitigate the impact on diet.

Peer Influence Peer pressure and social norms may influence food choices.

Choice: Building a supportive network, communicating personal dietary preferences and making independent choices that align with health goals can help navigate peer influence.

Chapter 4
Discovering the Power of Food

In the intricate tapestry of human existence, few elements wield as much influence over our well-being as the food we consume. Beyond mere sustenance, food has emerged as a catalyst for cultural, social and individual expressions. It is a source of nourishment that extends beyond the physiological, reaching into the realms of emotional, psychological and even spiritual dimensions. The journey of discovering the power of food is an exploration that transcends the kitchen and delves deep into the intricate connections between what we eat and how it shapes our lives.

The modern era has witnessed a paradigm shift in the way we perceive and interact with food. No longer confined to the basic necessities of survival, food has evolved into a realm where taste, texture and presentation are elevated to an art form. Simultaneously, an increasing awareness of the profound impact of our dietary choices on health and well-being has prompted a reevaluation of our relationship with food. Discovering the power of food is not just about satisfying our taste buds; it is about unlocking the potential of nutrition as a means to foster vitality, longevity and holistic wellness.

This exploration covers various aspects of our existence, from the physiological effects of different nutrients on our bodies to the cultural and historical significance of our culinary traditions.

Moreover, the power of food extends to social structures, bringing people from different backgrounds together through shared meals, rituals and celebrations.

Language has the ability to bridge gaps, create bonds and serve as a universal language that transcends cultural and linguistic barriers.

As we embark on this journey of discovery, we uncover the secrets of superfoods, explore the complex relationship between diet and mental health and delve into the cultural fabrics that connect the world's diverse cuisines.

The power of food is not limited to the plate. It extends to the decisions we make, the communities we build and the impact we have on the planet. We invite you to join us on this quest to unlock the potential of food beyond immediate taste pleasure.

Discovering the power of food is recognizing the deep and diverse role that what we eat plays in shaping our lives and, in turn, the world around us. The power of food goes far beyond basic provision. It plays an important role in our physical health, mental health and even cultural and social aspects of life.

Here are some ways food can do that:

Dietary Effects: Dietary Effects refers to the effect that dietary habits have on a person's health and well-being. A balanced and nutritious diet is essential for maintaining proper body function, supporting growth and development and preventing various health problems. The most important aspects of the nutritional effect of a diet are:

Macronutrients: Carbohydrates, proteins and fats are essential macronutrients that provide energy and play important roles in metabolic processes.

Micronutrients: Vitamins and minerals are micronutrients required for a variety of physiological functions, including immune support, bone health and enzyme activation.

Calorie intake: The balance between calorie intake and energy expenditure is critical to weight management and overall health.

Nutrient Density: Choosing nutritious foods ensures that your body receives essential nutrients without ingesting excess calories.

Hydration: Proper diet includes adequate fluid intake. This is important for digestion, nutrient absorption and overall health.

Impact on chronic diseases: Diet can influence the risk of chronic **diseases** such as cardiovascular disease, diabetes and obesity.

Gut Health: A diet rich in fiber supports gut health and has a positive effect on digestion and the microbiome.

Long-term effects: Consistent adherence to a balanced diet contributes to long-term health, prevents deficiency symptoms and promotes overall well-being.

Physical Health: Food provides essential nutrients such as vitamins, minerals, proteins, fats and carbohydrates that are essential for the proper functioning of our bodies. A balanced diet supports growth, development and overall health.

Disease Prevention: Certain foods are associated with preventing or reducing the risk of various diseases. For example, a diet high in fruits and vegetables reduces the risk of heart disease and foods high in antioxidants can help prevent certain types of cancer.

Mental Health: Brain Function: The brain requires a variety of nutrients to function optimally. Omega-3 fatty acids found in fish are associated with improved cognitive function and better mental health.

Mood and Emotions: Some foods can affect your mood and emotions because they affect the production of neurotransmitters.

For example, serotonin, a neurotransmitter that contributes to well-being, is influenced by the amino acid tryptophan found in certain foods.

Cultural Significance: Traditions and Rituals: Food often plays a central role in cultural traditions and rituals. Special dishes are prepared for celebrations, religious ceremonies and family gatherings, creating a sense of identity and connection.

Culinary Heritage: Different regions have unique culinary traditions that reflect local culture, history and available ingredients. Exploring and preserving this food tradition can foster a sense of pride and community.

Social Connect: Sharing and Connecting Food provides an opportunity to socialize, connect and share experiences. Eating together promotes communication and strengthens relationships with family and friends.

Culinary Experiences: **Exploring** different cuisines and culinary experiences brings people together, creating shared memories and a sense of togetherness.

Environmental Impact: Sustainable Choices: Our food choices can impact the environment. Choosing foods that are locally sourced, seasonal and sustainably produced helps protect the environment and reduce **your** carbon footprint

Economic Impact: Food Industry: The production, distribution and consumption of food has significant economic impacts. The food industry creates jobs, drives innovation and contributes to economic growth in many regions.

Understanding the power of food requires recognizing its diverse role in our lives, including not only nutrition and health, but also culture, social dynamics and environmental sustainability.

Chapter 5
Navigating Dietary Restrictions

Living with dietary restrictions can be challenging, but it can also be an opportunity for growth and creativity. This chapter covers my experiences with food allergies, intolerances, or medical conditions that required dietary adjustments. We discuss the emotional and practical aspects of managing these limitations while still enjoying delicious food.

Living with dietary restrictions is certainly difficult, but with a positive attitude and creativity, it is possible to successfully overcome these limitations. **Here are some tips for dealing with dietary restrictions:**

Get Educated: Learn more about the specific dietary restrictions you're struggling with.

Understand which foods are safe and which foods to avoid: This knowledge allows for informed decision-making and reduces the risk of accidental ingestion. Plan ahead because planning is key when you have dietary restrictions.

Study Menus and Product Labels: before going to a restaurant or store, study menus and product labels to find the right options. This will help you avoid last-minute stress and ensure you get a safe and enjoyable meal.

Cook at Home: Preparing your own meals makes it much easier to control the ingredients in your meals. Try new recipes and cooking techniques to make your meals interesting. There are many online resources and cookbooks that address specific dietary restrictions.

Communicate Clearly: Whether you're eating out, attending a social event, or staying with friends or family, be clear about your dietary restrictions. Please feel free to ask us any questions about materials or how to make them. Most people are understanding and willing to adapt.

Explore Alternative Ingredients: There are often alternative ingredients that can be used in place of ingredients that should be avoided. For example, if you follow a gluten-free diet, consider using almond or coconut flour when baking bread. By experimenting with different alternatives, you're likely to find one that's both delicious and filling.

Stock up on safe snacks: Stocking up on safe snacks can be a lifesaver, especially when you're on the go. Stock up on snacks that meet your dietary restrictions to avoid compromises due to hunger.

Build a support system: Share your dietary restrictions with friends and family so they can better understand your needs. A support system can provide emotional support and make social situations more comfortable.

Stay Positive: Focus on the foods you can enjoy and not the foods you should avoid.
Take the opportunity to explore new cuisines and discover delicious dishes within your dietary restrictions.

Read the Label Carefully: Read the label carefully when purchasing packaged foods. Food manufacturers may change their ingredients or manufacturing methods, so it's important to stay alert. Look for certifications that prove the product meets your nutritional needs.

Talk to a Professional: If you have health-related dietary restrictions, consider talking to a registered dietitian or health care professional. They will provide you with personalized advice to ensure you are meeting your nutritional needs while adhering to your dietary restrictions.

Remember that dealing with dietary restrictions is a journey of self-discovery and adaptation. With time and effort, you can develop a repertoire of delicious, filling meals that meet your specific nutritional needs.

Chapter 6
Finding Balance

In the complex dance of life, we often find ourselves caught between the temptations of pleasure and the demands of unwavering discipline. Finding the right balance between these two forces is a delicate art that requires introspection, self-awareness and a deep understanding of our desires and aspirations. In a world where temptations and obligations constantly bombard us, finding balance can be a journey of self-discovery and resilience. Harmony Within: Navigating the fine line between indulgence and discipline invites you on a transformative exploration of the complex interplay between pleasure and restraint.

This chapter didn't dictates rules of behavior in life, but a thoughtful guide that encourages you to embrace the beauty of balance. Through insightful reflections, practical exercises and real-life anecdotes, we embark on a quest to understand the dynamics of patience and discipline, uncovering the layers that define our choices and shape our destiny. How can we navigate the oceans of abundance without losing sight of our goals?

How can discipline increase our joy instead of suppressing it? These questions are a compass that guides us through the chapters, each of which unravels an aspect of the complex web of harmonious living. Whether you're seeking a healthier relationship with your habits, seeking personal growth, or simply improving your overall well-being, Harmony Within has the wisdom to illuminate your path.

Here are some tips to help you find that balance.

Set realistic goals: Set achievable short-term and long-term goals for your health and well-being. This will help you stay focused without getting overwhelmed.

Get some exercise: Enjoy snacks and fun in moderation. Treating yourself once in a while can help you avoid feelings of deprivation and maintain an overall healthy lifestyle.

Maintain a Balanced Diet: Include a variety of nutritious foods in your diet. This allows you to enjoy your favorite foods in moderation while ensuring you're getting essential vitamins, minerals and other nutrients.

Listen to your body: Pay attention to your hunger and fullness signals. Eat when you're hungry and stop when you're full. This helps prevent overeating and promotes a healthier relationship with food.

Plan Your Splurges: Plan ahead instead of impulsively splurging. Once you know you're getting a treat, it's easier to continue making healthier choices the rest of the time.

Get some physical activity: Regular exercise is an important part of a healthy lifestyle. Find activities you enjoy and make staying active fun rather than a chore.

Practice mindful eating: Be sure to attend mealtimes. Avoid distractions like screens and enjoy every bite. This will help you enjoy your food more and be more aware of your body's hunger and satiety signals.

Establish a Routine: Create a routine that includes regular meals, snacks and physical activity. Having a consistent schedule will make it easier to maintain a healthy lifestyle.

Stay hydrated: Drinking enough water is essential to your overall health. Feeling hungry may actually be a sign of dehydration. Make sure to stay hydrated throughout the day.

Forgive yourself: Don't be too hard on yourself if you overdo it or skip training. Acknowledge it, learn from it and move on. Guilt and stress can affect your overall health. Remember that finding balance is an ongoing process and its okay to adjust your approach as needed.

Chapter 7
The Joy of Cooking and Sharing

This chapter describes the joy of cooking healthy meals and sharing them with friends and family. I talk about my favorite recipes, meal planning tips and the satisfaction of nourishing others through food. I would like to emphasize the value of community support and note that it has played an important role in my journey. That's a great topic for a chapter! "Sharing the Love" emphasizes the positive aspects of cooking and how it creates connections and fosters a sense of community beyond the kitchen.

Here are some ideas and points you can consider when cooking healthy meals and sharing joy:

Cooking as an Expression of Love: Reinforces the idea that preparing food is a tangible way to demonstrate love and care for others. Discuss the joy and satisfaction that comes from making an effort to create something special for someone you love.

Gathering Experiences: Discover the communal side of sharing meals with others, including family dinners, potlucks and social gatherings. Share a personal story or anecdote about a memorable meal you shared with friends or family.

Healthy and Nutritious Eating: Emphasizes the importance of preparing nutritious and balanced meals to promote good health. Contains tips and recipes for creating delicious, healthy meals that everyone can enjoy.

Building Traditions: Discuss the role of cooking in building family traditions and the sense of continuity it provides. Encourages readers to start their own culinary traditions, whether it's a weekly family meal or an annual get-together.

Cook together: Discover the benefits of involving friends and family in the cooking process. Share ideas for cooking activities you can do together to have fun and bond.

Share Recipe: Encourage readers to share their favorite recipes with friends and family. Add a collection of recipes that are not only healthy, but also easy to share and make together.

Cooking Memories: Recall your precious memories about food and cooking. Encourages readers to create their own culinary memories and celebrate the moments that happen at the dinner table. The Gift of Food: Discuss the idea of giving the gift of a home-cooked meal, emphasizing thoughtfulness and a personal touch.
Share ideas for wrapping and giving food gifts with love.

Cultural Connections: Discover how cooking and sharing food can bridge cultural differences and create understanding. Highlights a variety of recipes highlighting different culinary traditions.

Cooking Classes and Workshops: Offer cooking classes and workshops to teach people how to make healthy and delicious meals. Focus on simple recipes using fresh, whole ingredients.

Online Cooking Videos and Tutorials: Create cooking videos and share them on platforms like YouTube and social media. Make it attractive and easy to understand and highlight the benefits of a balanced diet.

Community Cooking Event: Organize a community cooking event where people can come together to cook and enjoy a shared meal. This creates a sense of community and promotes a healthy culinary culture.

Collaborate with a Nutritionist: Work with a nutritionist or nutritionist to provide comprehensive information about healthy eating habits. This includes the nutritional value of different foods, portion control, meal planning and more.

Recipe Sharing Platform: Create or join online forums and platforms where people can share their favorite healthy recipes. Encourage discussion of nutrition tips and tricks.

Chapter 8

Power of Self-Compassion and Resilience

With the constant pursuit of health and wellness in our busy modern lives, our eating habits are an important pillar that influences our overall well-being. The journey to a healthier lifestyle is often full of challenges and can seem difficult at times. But the realm of self-compassion and resilience holds deep secrets. It is a transformative force that can change not only the way we eat, but also the nature of our well-being.

In this insightful chapter, "The Power of Self-Compassion and Resilience in Transforming Nutritional Habits for Lasting Happiness," It delves into the complex interplay between passion and the heart.

Nutritional choices form the basis of our daily lives. Based on the latest research in psychology, nutrition and holistic health, this book shows how self-compassion and resilience can have a huge impact on our relationship with food and, in turn, our overall health. As we embark on this chapter, we will unravel the threads that connect our inner well-being to the decisions we make at the dinner table.

The following pages provide not only a guide to healthier eating habits, but also a holistic approach that considers the complex dynamics between mind, body and nutrition. Through anecdotes, science and practical strategies, Nourish Your Soul harnesses self-compassion as a powerful tool to cultivate resilience that not only endures the challenges of change, but turns them into opportunities for growth.

I encourage you to get ready to discover the transformative potential at the intersection of self-compassion and resilience, a dynamic force that can free you from the shackles of unhealthy eating and lead you to a life where happiness is more than just a goal. Join us on this fascinating journey as we uncover the secrets of nourishing your soul through the restorative power of self-compassion and food.

Self-compassion and resilience when it comes to your eating habits can have a huge impact on your overall well-being.

Here's how:

Reduce stress and emotional eating: Self-compassion means treating yourself with kindness and understanding. When you make a nutritional mistake or face a challenge, self-compassion allows you to respond with self-kindness rather than self-criticism. Resilience allows you to bounce back from setbacks and reduces the likelihood of seeking emotional comfort through food during stressful times.

Healthy Relationship with Food: Self-compassion promotes a positive attitude towards yourself, including your body and diet. This allows you to be more mindful and in tune with your body's needs, giving you a healthier relationship with food. Resilience helps you stay true to your nutritional goals despite occasional setbacks, promoting a long-term, sustainable approach to healthy eating.

Increased Motivation: Self-compassion is linked to intrinsic motivation. When you approach dietary changes with self-compassion, you're more likely to be motivated by a desire for self-improvement and well-being, rather than external pressure or criticism. If you are resilient, setbacks will not affect your motivation. Instead, view challenges as opportunities to learn and grow and stay positive about your nutrition journey.

Mindful Eating: Both self-compassion and resilience contribute to mindfulness.

Being present in the moment and paying attention to your body's hunger and fullness signals will result in a more conscious and satisfying eating experience. Resilience helps you cope with the prevalence of unhealthy foods and allows you to make prudent decisions even in difficult environments.

Long-term success: Self-compassion and resilience contribute to a more sustainable approach to dietary change. Rather than being defeated by setbacks, you can adapt and persevere through hardships. Resilience allows you to see nutritional mistakes as opportunities for growth rather than failures, making you more likely to stick to your long-term goals.

Emotion Regulation: Self-compassion provides a framework for dealing with negative emotions without resorting to unhealthy coping mechanisms such as emotional eating. Resilience helps you weather the ups and downs of your nutrition journey and prevents emotional setbacks from leading to a complete abandonment of healthy habits. Incorporating self-compassion and resilience into your approach to dietary change can create a more positive and sustainable relationship with food, ultimately contributing to your overall health and well-being.

Conclusion

In conclusion, my Diet my Happiness goes beyond traditional nutritional approaches and serves as a comprehensive guide that addresses the complex relationships between nutrition, well-being and overall well-being. Through careful consideration of scientific research, personal anecdotes and practical advice, the author crafts a compelling story that allows readers to make informed decisions about their eating habits and lifestyle.

This book emphasizes that nutrition has a huge impact not only on physical health, but also on mental and emotional well-being. She advocates for a holistic approach that considers individual needs, preferences and cultural influences, recognizing that one-size-fits-all solutions are not sufficient in the complex area of nutrition and well-being.

Additionally, the author emphasize the importance of fostering a positive relationship with food, moving away from restrictive approaches and developing a mindset that promotes mindful eating. By combining scientific discoveries with relatable stories, Diet, Health and Happiness successfully bridges the gap between academic knowledge and practical application, making information accessible and practical for readers from all walks of life.

As readers scroll through the pages, they'll not only gain a better understanding of nutrition, but they'll also be inspired to embark on a transformational journey to a healthier, happier life. This book challenges conventional wisdom, encourages critical thinking and gives readers the tools they need to take control of their own happiness.

Ultimately, my Diet my Happiness is a beacon of enlightenment in the crowded landscape of health literature, providing a balanced and informative look at the complex interplay between diet, health and the pursuit of happiness. It not only provides readers with a wealth of knowledge, but also the motivation and confidence to pursue a personal path to optimal health.